INCREASING THE SUPPLY
OF MEDICAL PERSONNEL

Evaluative Studies

This series of studies seeks to bring about greater understanding and promote continuing review of the activities and functions of the federal government. Each study focuses on a specific program, evaluating its cost and efficiency, the extent to which it achieves its objectives, and the major alternative means—public and private—for reaching those objectives. Yale Brozen, professor of economics at the University of Chicago and an adjunct scholar of the American Enterprise Institute for Public Policy Research, is the director of the program.

INCREASING THE SUPPLY OF MEDICAL PERSONNEL

Needs and alternatives

Charles T. Stewart, Jr.
Corazon M. Siddayao

American Enterprise Institute for Public Policy Research
Washington, D. C.

Charles T. Stewart, Jr. is professor of economics at The George Washington University.

Corazon M. Siddayao is a teaching fellow in the department of economics at The George Washington University.

ISBN 0-8447-3097-1

Evaluative Studies 6, March 1973

Library of Congress Catalog Card No. L.C. 73-77435

Printed in the United States of America

CONTENTS

1783156

INTRODUCTION

In 1963 the federal government initiated direct assistance to increase the supply of health care manpower. Since then, there has been a continuing health manpower shortage, resulting in a series of congressional acts, the most recent of which are the Comprehensive Manpower Training Act and the Nurse Training Act of 1971.

The shortage of medical manpower was aggravated by increased demand produced by other federal programs, specifically Medicare and Medicaid. These programs reduced the effective price of medical care for persons who had previously been able to afford only emergency care. This led to an increased demand for nonemergency care. Since measures to increase supply work only with a time lag, the gap between supply and demand worsened in the later 1960s.

This paper considers medical personnel shortages, especially the shortage of physicians, and the different ways to alleviate these shortages. Chapter I gives a brief history (1963-1972) of legislation intended to increase medical manpower supply. Chapter II discusses the causes of the shortage, analyzing the elements affecting demand for medical care in recent years and the elements affecting supply. Chapter III analyzes the possible need for federal subsidies. It points out the short-term nature of the problem and the long-term effects of federal solutions. It also discusses the maldistribution in the supply of medical manpower by geographical area and among specialties. Chapter IV outlines ways of increasing the productivity of present supply through more efficient utilization. Chapter V questions the priority placed on manpower supply in the struggle to upgrade the level of national health, and suggests alternative courses of action.

1

CHAPTER I

FEDERAL PROGRAMS FOR MEDICAL MANPOWER TRAINING

Considerable attention has been directed toward the problem of increasing health care services in the United States. In recent years, government programs have played a key role in the medical sector, bearing part of the cost of services and subsidizing the training of health personnel.

The federal government first gave direct assistance aimed at enlarging the supply of medical manpower with the Health Professions Education Act of 1963 (P.L. 88-129). It provided a three-year program of matching grants, beginning with fiscal year 1964, for construction and improvement of schools for physicians, dentists, pharmacists, optometrists, podiatrists, nurses and "professional public health personnel." It also provided a six-year program of loans to students pursuing doctoral degrees in medicine, dentistry, and osteopathy.

The Nurse Training Act of 1964 (P.L. 88-581) authorized matching grants for construction, expansion, and rehabilitation of nursing schools and for curriculum improvements for the years 1966 through 1969. Assistance to student optometrists was added by P.L. 88-654 in 1964. The Health Professions Educational Assistance Amendments (P.L. 89-290 in 1965) set up a system of scholarships. In addition, it included a program of educational improvement grants to stimulate enrollment in medical and paramedical schools and to improve the quality of education in these schools for the fiscal years 1968 and 1969. These amendments included a "forgiveness" principle for loans to students who practiced in an underserved area following graduation. The Allied Health Professions Personnel Training Act (P.L. 89-751 of 1966), which further amended the 1963 legislation, allowed a cancellation of 15 percent a year, up to 100 percent of the loan and interest, for a physician who practiced in a low-income rural area designated by the secretary of Health, Education and Welfare. It provided for expanding and improving the training of semiprofessional manpower, and further broadened the 1963 legislation.

The Health Manpower Act of 1968 (P.L. 90-490) extended federal support, beginning with fiscal year 1970, and imposed specific restrictions on how federal funds would be spent. Besides amending the various provisions of the 1963 legislation and four other laws (including the Nurse Training Act of 1964 and the Allied Health Professions Personnel Training Act of 1966), it included incentives to encourage medical and nursing schools to increase their enrollments. It enlarged the scholarship and loan programs. It increased the federal share in construction costs for financially needy schools, set up a scheme to reward schools according to increases in enrollment, and provided special grants for innovative curricula which would expand and improve manpower supply.[1]

Two laws enacted in 1971, the Comprehensive Health Manpower Training Act (P.L. 92-157) and the Nurse Training Act (P.L. 92-158) are intended primarily to accelerate the increase in the number of medical personnel. These acts cover assistance grants to schools of medicine, osteopathy, dentistry, and nursing, including bonus grants for increasing enrollments by 5 percent and for graduating doctors in less than four years. There are also grants for the training of other health professionals. Public Law 92-157 covers a wide range of programs dealing with the problems of shortages of medical personnel—not only shortages in the aggregate but shortages through maldistribution. To improve distribution of health care, it provides for incentives to attract physicians to currently underserved areas [2] and special grants to increase the number of graduates in certain fields, such as family medicine.[3] The law also provides for scholarships and loans to U.S. citizens enrolled in foreign medical schools.[4]

The Uniformed Services Health Professions Revitalization Act of 1972 (P.L. 92-426) authorizes a special school of medicine exclusively for the armed forces and establishes scholarships at existing medical schools to train military doctors. The measure is intended to meet the problem of providing medical attention for members of the armed forces and their dependents that will result from the expected decreased supply of military doctors when the draft for doctors ends.

The manpower training acts were followed by significant increases in the number of physicians, dentists, and nurses entering the field annually. In 1971 the number of graduating physicians was

4

3 percent greater than in 1963, and enrollments in schools of medicine and osteopathy were up by 30 percent over the same period. Sixteen new schools of medicine and osteopathy opened in the 1960s, compared with six in the 1950s and two in the 1940s. The annual number of dentistry graduates has increased by 18 percent since 1963 and nursing graduates by 24 percent since the enactment of the Nurse Training Act in 1964.[5] The presumption is that the earlier medical manpower training acts were instrumental in bringing about this substantial increase in training capacity and output of medical personnel, although increases began before they were enacted, and that the 1971 legislation will result in a further increase. The issues to be discussed in the following chapters are the extent of the shortage of medical personnel, and the need and desirability of the new federal subsidies to eliminate it.

CHAPTER II

CAUSES OF THE SHORTAGE

Whether there is a need for additional medical personnel depends on the demand for and supply of medical services. The current shortage was brought about by an unprecedented increase in the demand for medical care, particularly in the late 1960s, in great part because of Medicare, Medicaid, and the growth in private third party payments. The demand pressure was not met by a parallel supply response. Not only is there a time lag in training and graduating personnel, especially doctors whose training usually requires at least five years beyond the bachelor's degree,[1] but also a special problem in the nature of the demand for and supply of medical care itself.

Demand for Medical Care

The demand for medical care is derived from the final demand for good health. Demand usually cannot be measured directly. It is observed from data that measure rates of utilization resulting from the interplay of demand and supply. In an analysis of the demand for medical care, both factors have to be taken into account. To some extent in the medical field, supply creates its own demand.

Factors Affecting Demand for Medical Care. The major determinants of demand for medical care can be put into two groups. First, there are those that influence ability to purchase care—income, price of medical care and other goods, and health insurance coverage and philanthropy, whether government or private. Second, there are those that influence consumer preferences and choices—family size, age, sex, culture characteristics, education, technology, geographical location, and availability of physicians.[2]

Empirical studies have shown that families with higher incomes have higher expenditures on medical care.[3] It has also been suggested that expenditures are related to permanent rather than to current income (i.e., they are fairly independent of fluctuations in income). The income-expenditure relationship is of course two-way: demand for health services is a function of the health of the individual, and the health of the individual could at some income levels be directly related to his income. The lowest income groups are more likely to have poor nutrition and inappropriate health habits, and may require health attention more frequently than higher income groups. On the other hand, demand for nonemergency medical care is strongly influenced by level of income. In the absence of third party payments or philanthropy, lower income means, other things being equal, smaller medical expenditures and postponement of all but emergency care.

The price of medical care influences the demand for medical care. However, for certain types of medical care, the magnitude of this effect is small. Also, it is reduced by insurance and philanthropy, which lower the effective price of the care.

One approach toward measuring the need for more medical personnel in the long run is the forecasting of the behavior of demand for medical care as incomes increase and as prices change. Increases in income tend to raise, whereas increases in price tend to reduce, the amount demanded.

Various studies indicate that the income elasticity of demand for medical care is well below unity.[4] Thus if prices remain unchanged, expenditures on medical care would be a declining proportion of income.[5] Price elasticity of demand has been found to be very low; for physician visits it is estimated at 0.2.[6] But elasticities vary widely from one type of service to another. The demand for emergency care is highly inelastic, insensitive to income or price. But when medical care is not a matter of life and death, but is postponable or even dispensable, people do consider price and their pocketbooks. It is, to summarize, the combination of the growth in third party payments and of the rise in prices, rather than growing incomes, that explains the increasing share of income spent on medical care in recent years and for the years ahead.

Demand for medical care varies with age and sex. The number of physician visits is higher for the young (under five years) and the old (65 and over) than for others, and higher for females than for males.[7] Women in the child-bearing age consume more medical care (of a specific type) than other women. That these are the people

8

who also have more time to spare to seek medical care also influences their use of medical services.

Marital status likewise affects demand. A single person living alone may seek hospital care for an illness which for a person living with his family would only mean care at home. Family structure, which is connected with the size of household, affects the demand for medical services and in particular for hospitalization and other institutionalized care. The small nuclear family may not be able to nurse a sick member, and must send him to a hospital. An extended family, or even a large nuclear family, is more likely to accommodate the needs of the sick within the framework of its work and school duties. Likewise, care for the aged is transferred from family to nursing home or similar institution in an urban society where nuclear families dominate. Social change in America has contributed to the increase in demand for institutionalized medical care.

Cultural differences affect the use of physician services. According to one study, the utilization rate of physician services by nonwhites was 70 percent of that by whites of the same income level.[8] This pattern was not expected to remain unchanged, and in fact utilization rates have risen. Other studies point out the effect of cultural differences on demand for health care. States with high proportions of Scandinavians have high levels of health;[9] immigrant Jews, in spite of extreme poverty, have very low infant mortality; Japanese children in California have low accident rates;[10] and New York Jews have a high incidence of coronary heart disease.[11]

The relationship of education to demand for medical care is complex. Since the level of education is often related to the level of income, it is difficult to separate the effects of the two. Education may increase demand through greater awareness of medical and health needs. On the other hand, greater education could mean better living habits and fewer illnesses, which would lower expenditures for certain types of medical attention.

Changes in medical knowledge and technology raise the expectations of consumers that medical services will bring them greater benefits and tend to increase demand. New services become available for previously untreatable conditions (as, for example, cornea transplants), and these services generate their own demand. Probably more than in earlier days, the adage that "an ounce of prevention is worth a pound of cure" moves people to seek preventive care.

Changes in technology may also increase the use of physician services if the new technology is "physician-intensive." Since 1956, most advances in medical technology (for example, renal dialysis, cancer chemotherapy, open heart surgery), though producing only marginal improvements in general health indices, have required large inputs of physician time and increased hospital use. In contrast, the technological advances of the 1940s, such as antibiotics, economized on physician and hospital services.[12]

Demand is affected to a large extent by the medical profession itself. Observers seem to agree that the demand side of the medical care market is imperfect.[13] Consumers often are not in a position to assess the quality and character of the medical services they need and the range of alternatives open. They rely on the judgment of the doctor (the seller) who determines the mix of medical services, tells them when to come back to see him, who else to see, what tests to take, what operation to have, what medicines to take, even what hospital to use. Frequently demand is what the profession decides that a person needs, rather than the result of a rational calculation by the consumer based on what he wants and can afford, and on his awareness of alternatives and consequences.[14]

Scientific standards are uncertain and the subject of frequent debate. In many cases, the comparative effectiveness of alternatives is all that is taken into consideration: marginal benefits relative to costs per unit of service are not often weighed before therapeutic procedures are recommended.[15] Especially when there is insurance coverage, the economic circumstances of the patient are not taken into consideration. The physician provides the best care technologically possible at any cost, providing the patient or some third party is willing to pay for it. This policy may be explained in part by medical ethics and tradition, in part by a fear of malpractice suits, in part perhaps by other factors.

The number of physicians available also influences the demand for and utilization of medical care. In normal markets, an excess supply depresses prices, and a greater number of physicians would tend to lower the price of physician's services. The market for physician's services does not however operate as traditional theory suggests. Pricing in the physician care market does not systematically vary with supply; rather, demand for physician's services adjusts to the availability of physicians. Prices do not fall, but when there is a sufficient number of physicians available, the costs of waiting and travel decline, which encourages greater use of physician's services. It is possible that, with an increase in the number of doctors, quality of medical services rises, and cost per unit of service falls, even though fees do not fall.

More important, however, when there is an abundance of physicians in a given geographical area or field of specialization, care may be prescribed which is not medically indicated (for example, unnecessary surgery) or of only marginal importance (for example, numerous postoperative visits). Since the consumer is in no position independently to assess his requirements, his demand is related to the availability of physician's services. On the other hand, where physicians are scarce and where patients may have a long wait to get service, they may handle their minor complaints themselves. The physician will ration his services so that only those really needed are given.

The significance of the physician's discretionary influence cannot be overstressed. To the extent that physicians can influence the demand for medical care, attempts to relieve shortages by increasing the supply of medical personnel (and facilities) are self-defeating.

Growth of Demand in Recent Years. The rise in demand for medical care can be observed from the growth in expenditures on medical care. Table 1 shows changes in expenditures over the years.

During the period from fiscal year 1950 to fiscal year 1971, per-capita expenditures in current dollars rose from $78 to $358. Per-capita expenditures on health in constant dollars (using the consumer price index deflator, see Table 2) rose 170 percent. In terms of the medical care component of the price index, the growth in actual care received per capita was 90 percent.

Total national health expenditures in current dollars rose $63 billion, or 525 percent from the 1950 level.[16] In constant dollars, the rise was 270 percent. In real terms (using the medical services component rather than the consumer price index deflator), the growth in expenditures showed a 160 percent increase in medical care received.[17]

In terms of the proportion of GNP spent on health care services, the growth of expenditures during the period 1965-1971 exceeded that of any earlier period (see Table 1). In 1970 and 1971, it was 54 and 60 percent, respectively, above the 1950 level.

The Role of Third Party Payments in Demand Growth. A major factor in the growth in demand for medical care has been the growth in third party payments.[18] In the 1950s private health insurance grew substantially. By fiscal year 1960, third parties paid 45 percent of the personal health care bill.[19] Private health insurance paid 21 percent of the total (up from 7 percent in fiscal year 1950), and government paid 22 percent of the total.[20]

The pattern changed in 1966 with the implementation of the 1965 Social Security Amendments (Medicare and Medicaid). Under Medicare, government-funded and voluntary medical insurance bene-

Table 1

NATIONAL HEALTH EXPENDITURES, BY SOURCE OF FUNDS AND AS PERCENT OF GNP SELECTED YEARS 1950 THROUGH 1971

Fiscal Year	Gross National Product (billions)	National Health Expenditures						
		Total			Private		Public	
		Amount (millions)	Per capita	Percent of GNP	Amount (millions)	Percent of total	Amount (millions)	Percent of total
1949-50	$ 263.4	$12,028	$ 78.35	4.6	$ 8,962	74.5	$ 3,065	25.5
1954-55	379.7	17,330	103.76	4.6	12,909	74.5	4,420	25.5
1959-60	495.6	25,857	141.64	5.2	19,460	75.3	6,395	24.7
1964-65	655.6	38,892	197.81	5.9	29,357	75.5	9,535	24.5
1965-66	718.5	42,109	211.64	5.9	31,279	74.3	10,830	25.7
1966-67	771.4	47,860	237.93	6.2	32,037	66.9	15,823	33.1
1967-68	827.0	53,563	263.49	6.5	33,523	62.6	20,040	37.4
1968-69	898.4	59,939	292.01	6.7	37,004	61.7	22,935	38.3
1969-70	953.2	67,770	326.78	7.1	42,738	63.1	25,032	36.9
1970-71	1,008.5	75,012	358.05	7.4	46,548	62.1	28,463	37.9

Source: Derived from Dorothy P. Rice and Barbara S. Cooper, "National Health Expenditures, 1929-1971," in Social Security Administration, Social Security Bulletin, January 1972, Table 1, p. 5.

12

Table 2

INDICES OF MEDICAL CARE PRICES
(1967 = 100)

Year	Consumer Price Index		Professional Services (selected items)		Hospital Daily Charges
	All items	Medical care[a]	Physician's fees	Dentist's fees	
1950	72.1	53.7	55.2	63.9	28.9
1955	80.2	64.8	65.4	73.0	41.5
1960	88.7	79.1	77.0	82.1	56.3
1965	94.5	89.5	88.3	92.2	76.6
1966	97.2	93.4	93.4	95.2	84.0
1967	100.0	100.0	100.0	100.0	100.0
1968	104.2	106.1	105.6	105.5	113.2
1969	109.8	113.4	112.9	112.9	127.9
1970	116.3	120.6	121.4	119.4	143.9
1971	121.3	128.4	129.8	127.0	160.8

a Medical care component includes drugs and prescriptions, professional services for obstetrical cases, tonsillectomies, adenoidectomies, optometric examination and eyeglasses, in addition to physician's fees and dentist's fees.

Source: U.S. Bureau of the Census, *Statistical Abstract of the United States, 1972* (Washington: U.S. Government Printing Office, 1972), Tables 90 and 565.

fits were provided to elderly people, 65 and over.[21] Medicaid provided federally aided state government health benefits and expanded health services to millions of low-income people not covered by Medicare. Government became the source of more than half of third party payments after 1966. Third party payments rose from 47 percent of personal health care expenditures in 1965 to 63 percent in 1971 (see Table 3).

Widespread insurance coverage increases the demand for medical care by reducing the out-of-pocket expense paid by the consumer. The decision of the consumer is distorted by the fact that he does not bear the full burden of medical care while he does bear the full burden of other expenses. Medicare and Medicaid have had the same distorting impact.

Certain types of medical attention were demanded, even when not absolutely necessary, if they were covered by insurance. Many aged and low-income persons were receiving free medical care through free clinics or hospitals or charitable institutions before implementation of the program. The more liberal privileges under Medicare and Medicaid, however, allowed a great number of people to seek medical services they would have foregone because it was not paid for under previous programs.[22] An indication of this can

Table 3

PERCENTAGE DISTRIBUTION OF SOURCES
FOR PERSONAL HEALTH CARE EXPENDITURES
SELECTED YEARS 1950-1971

Fiscal Year	Direct Private Payments (1)	Third Party Payments		
		Private (2)	Public (3)	Total (2+3)
1949-50	68.3	11.5	20.2	31.7
1954-55	59.0	18.2	22.8	41.0
1959-60	55.3	23.0	21.7	44.7
1964-65	52.5	26.7	20.8	47.5
1965-66	51.5	26.7	21.8	48.5
1966-67	45.4	24.4	30.2	54.6
1967-68	40.8	24.2	35.0	59.2
1968-69	39.0	25.0	36.0	61.0
1969-70	39.0	26.0	35.0	61.0
1970-71	37.2	27.0	35.8	62.8

Source: Derived from Dorothy P. Rice and Barbara S. Cooper, "National Health Expenditures, 1929-1971," in Social Security Administration, *Social Security Bulletin,* January 1972, Table 5.

be found in the utilization of hospital facilities over the period 1965-1967. The average stay lengthened from 9.1 to 9.9 days. That increased third party coverage allowed people to stay longer than they did formerly can be inferred from observation of the statistics during the period of installation of Medicare and Medicaid.

There was already a shortage of medical personnel following the rapid growth of private insurance before the introduction of Medicare and Medicaid. Implementation of these programs increased demand further and worsened the shortage.

The Supply Response

In most sectors of the economy, the supply of goods and services is largely governed by the net return realized from their production as compared with the net returns realized from using the same resources elsewhere. These net returns depend in part on the relative demand for goods and services. Given the conditions where sellers are willing to supply certain goods and services and buyers want and are able to pay for these same goods and services, the market is cleared at the price equating demand and supply. Price serves a rationing function. The market pricing mechanism also applies to medical care services. Additional supplies are called forth in response to higher prices resulting from increased demand, although certain factors prevent this mechanism from working as conventional theory suggests.

Factors Affecting the Supply of Medical Care. The supply of medical care is affected (1) by the state of technology and organization affecting productivity, (2) by the number of medical personnel and the capacity of facilities, and (3) by the location of personnel and facilities relative to demand or need. The rate at which supply can be increased is influenced (1) by time lags in graduating personnel and building facilities, (2) by entry limitations to medical schools and the rate of attrition in such schools, (3) by licensing requirements for physicians, (4) by the rate of retirements and deaths in the profession, (5) by the returns to those supplying medical care, (6) by the capital market for medical facilities investment, (7) by locational decisions of physicians and auxiliary personnel, (8) by the existence of a vertical gap in the hierarchy of medical personnel,[23] (9) by the rate of introduction of new technology affecting productivity of medical personnel and facilities, and (10) by the rate of improvement in the organization of the delivery of medical care.

Imperfections in the medical care market exist on the supply side as well as on the demand side. In discussing the factors affecting demand we mentioned the unique role of the physician as decision maker in determining what medical goods and services the patient needs to have. Physicians are, for example, in a position to decide when a condition requires hospital confinement and how long a patient has to stay—a decision which affects the amounts of goods and services supplied.

To the extent this ability of supply to create its own demand exists, it frustrates attempts to relieve shortages by increasing supply. Moreover, other market imperfections restrict supply even in the presence of excess demand. There are monopolistic elements in the market. Entry is restricted not only through medical schools but also through licensing, certification, or membership requirements in professional societies.[24] Membership in county or state societies is sometimes necessary for the use of hospital facilities.[25]

The supply sector of medical care differs from that of ordinary goods and services insofar as the production of medical care is directed towards supplying medical "needs" rather than meeting monetary demands. This special character of the supply of medical care leads to investment decisions being made on the basis of estimates by the profession of the "needs" of society rather than on projected demand in the normal market sense. Many specialized health facilities (such as coronary care units and provision for open heart surgery) are built with "excess standby capacity" intended to meet emergencies with little balance between the probable extent of any probable emergency and the facilities provided.

Growth of Personnel and Facilities. The current shortage of doctors is sometimes traced to the closing of many medical schools early in the century as a result of the Flexner Report in 1910.[26] After the number of "Class A" schools reached 77 in 1933, it stayed at that figure for 15 years (except for 1943 when there were only 76). While the closings were well intentioned, it is at least arguable that the powers extended to organized medicine to maintain a high standard of medical education have been overused to limit supply for the economic self-interest of the group.[27] By exercising its power to certify schools and hospitals fit to educate and train doctors, the AMA reduced the number of medical schools in the United States from 160 in 1905 to 88 in 1920 and 76 in 1930.[28]

From 1934 to 1945, the schools turned out an average of 5,100 graduates a year. This allowed the profession to keep the aggregate ratio of doctors to population relatively unchanged over the years,[29] but did not allow for changing requirements resulting from advances in science and technology, nor for changing utilization resulting from changes in income and education, nor for changing patterns of delivery of health care and population.[30] The ratio has inched upward in recent years, because of the influx of foreign-trained physicians and the increase in annual graduates from American schools beginning in 1951. From an average of 5,100 graduates annually from 1934 to 1945, the number rose to an average of 6,800 graduates annually from 1953 to 1959 and 7,200 annually from 1960 to 1966.[31] By 1966 the schools were graduating 36 percent more doctors than they had graduated in 1950. By 1971, they were graduating 63 percent more.[32] The rapid increase in recent years was presumably a response to demand and to federal pressure to increase the supply of doctors.[33] But direct federal help did not begin until 1964, and with the inevitable lag of several years, did not influence the number of graduates before 1968.

The rate of withdrawal from the profession through death or retirement is placed at 5,000 to 6,000 per year.[34] To keep up with the growth of demand, the nation's supply of doctors had to be augmented by foreign sources. Table 4 shows the number of physicians and surgeons immigrating into the United States during the period from fiscal year 1949 to fiscal year 1970.[35] In 1969, 23 percent of licenses issued (2,307 of a total of 9,978) were to physicians originally coming from foreign schools.[36] During the period 1959 to 1969 the

Table 4

IMMIGRANT PHYSICIANS AND SURGEONS
FISCAL YEARS 1949-1970

Fiscal Year	Number	Fiscal Year	Number
1949	1,148	1960	1,574
1950	1,848	1961	1,683
1951	1,387	1962	1,797
1952	1,201	1963	2,093
1953	845	1964	2,249
1954	1,040	1965	2,012
1955	1,046	1966	2,549
1956	1,388	1967	3,325
1957	1,990	1968	3,060
1958	1,934	1969	2,756
1959	1,630	1970	3,155

Source: National Science Foundation, based on data of the Immigration and Naturalization Service, U.S. Department of Justice.

proportion of physicians on record with the American Medical Association who were graduates of foreign medical schools (most but not all being foreigners) rose from 8.6 percent to 18.4 percent.[37]

The increase in foreign-trained non-U.S. citizens entering the medical field may be assumed to result from the increased demand for medical personnel and the economic and professional attractiveness of a U.S. practice. In particular the growth of short-term hospitals not associated with medical schools provided a demand for foreign interns, residents, and staff. In 1971, there were 14,500 foreign-trained interns and residents in U.S. hospitals (most but not all of them foreigners).[38]

Present standards and quotas under which schools and hospitals operate are unnecessarily restrictive and probably even monopolistic. Restriction of entry into professional schools could be justified if there were a lack of qualified applicants. The evidence indicates no such lack. In fact, poor chances for admission may discourage qualified applicants who do not apply and go into other fields instead. The fact that the number of schools and graduates was kept at a constant level for a prolonged period in spite of growth in population, income, general education, and membership in other professions can only give rise to the suspicion of effective control of supply for reasons other than quality maintenance. It would be logical to expect a significant rise in the number of schools and graduates, considering the rise in the number of college graduates and in the levels of family income.

In the academic year 1933-34, 62.5 percent of applicants to medical schools were accepted. As the number of applicants increased, the proportion accepted declined steadily to 29.3 percent in 1949-50. In 1949, there were more than three applicants for each place in medical school. The ratio of applicants to those accepted declined slowly to 1.7 in 1960 and 1961 (reflecting in part a great temporary expansion of federal assistance to graduate education in other fields). The ratio rose to an average level of two applicants for every place during the period 1962 to 1969.[39] In 1972, it was estimated that nationwide approximately two-thirds of the applicants to medical schools and one-half the qualified applicants would be turned down.[40]

Another indication that the number of qualified applicants far exceeds the number accepted is the extraordinarily low number of admitted applicants who do not graduate. The percentage not graduating in four years, a low 4.4 percent in 1950, rose to a peak of 13.7 percent in 1961, then declined steadily to 6.7 percent in 1966.[41] To the writers' knowledge no other professional curriculum produces this high rate of successful completion. It may be concluded that a substantial expansion of medical school student enrollment is possible without sacrifice in quality and without student subsidies.

Licensing requirements (which cover length of education, course requirements, examinations, and so on) vary from state to state and thereby affect the mobility of supply. In fact, some of them are likely to inhibit present trends in medical education—trends such as program acceleration, blurring of premedical and medical boundaries, integration of instruction in basic and clinical sciences, and new patterns of medical care delivery (such as the expanded roles of paramedics).[42]

As shown in Table 5, growth of demand for medical services was accompanied by a growth of supply. The ratio of physicians in private practice to population decreased from 1950 to 1965. It rose in 1966 and 1967.[43] The decline from 1950 to 1965 was partly the result of increases in the relative importance of teaching, research, and other nonpatient care activities. In part, it was the result of the increase of salaried physicians in hospitals, including interns, residents, fellows, and regular full-time staff members.[44]

It may be noted that there has been a recent increase in nursing graduates also. More than 43,600 nurses were graduated in 1970, about 24 percent more than were graduated in 1964.[45] The number of registered nurses has increased from 282 per 100,000 population in 1960 to 345 per 100,000 in 1970.[46] As with doctors, a large portion of the increase came from foreign countries.

Table 5

RATIO OF HEALTH PERSONNEL AND FACILITIES TO POPULATION
SELECTED YEARS 1950-1970
(per 100,000 population)

Year	Physicians [a]		Nurses	Hospital Personnel[b]	Short-term Hospital Beds[c]
	Total	In private practice			
1950	149	109	249	697	333
1955	150	102	259	788	344
1960	148	98	282	888	355
1965	153	97	319	1,009	383
1966	156	98	313	1,077	393
1967	158	100	325	1,116	399
1968	NA	NA	331	1,156	404
1969	163	NA	338	1,205	410
1970	171	NA	345	1,245	411

a Doctors of medicine and osteopathy.

b Derived from Table 99 in *Statistical Abstract, 1971*, and Table 107 in *Statistical Abstract, 1972*, using resident population data in the same source.

c Derived from Table 89 in *Statistical Abstract, 1968*, and Table 107 in *Statistical Abstract, 1972*. Federal hospitals are excluded. The ratio of all hospital beds to population declined because of the sharp drop in psychiatric beds.

Source: *Statistical Abstract of the United States, 1967-1972* editions.

Rise in Medical Fees and Other Prices. Given a manpower shortage, and a supply of medical services that does not adjust quickly to price increases, the pressure of increased demand from Medicare and Medicaid has caused prices for medical care to rise faster than prices of other items (Table 2). The sharpest rises were in physicians' fees and hospital charges.

Physicians' fees. Calculations by Newhouse and Taylor show that while physicians' fees rose by an average annual rate of 3.2 percent during fiscal years 1961 to 1966, the rise in fiscal year 1967 was more than twice as great (7.5 percent).[47] The rate of increase slowed to 6.1 percent in fiscal year 1968 and rose again to 6.7 percent in fiscal year 1969.

During the eleven-year period 1959-1970, the median net income of physicians in private practice rose by 88 percent (from $22,100 to $41,500).[48] While the mean income of general practitioners rose by 22.1 percent during the five-year period 1959-1964, it rose by 25.0 percent in the two-year period 1965-1967 (following Medicare and Medicaid), and by nearly 50 percent during the five-year period

1965-1970. Internists' mean income rose by 14.7 percent during the five-year period 1959-1964, by 17.3 percent during the two-year period 1965-1967, and by 48.8 percent during the five-year period 1965-1970. The highest growth in income was among general practitioners, whose median net earnings rose by 87 percent (from $20,000 in 1959 to $37,400 in 1970), and the lowest was among general surgeons (this lowest rate was 61 percent), making clear the shortage of general practitioners and the relative oversupply of general surgeons—even though general surgeons had a median income of $45,000 in 1970. The highest median earnings in 1970 were those of obstetrician-gynecologists ($47,050); the rate of growth was 68.6 percent or the second lowest. Internists ranked third in median income with $41,250 but the growth of their income was 85 percent—almost as high as that of general practitioners[49] (see Appendix Table 3).

The rise in earnings and in medical costs is not entirely explained by the increase in stated fees. There is some evidence that insurance results in higher fees for the same service,[50] but the major effect came from Medicare. Because the government guaranteed the payment of "customary fees," doctors who formerly charged the aged and poor less no longer found it necessary to do so. Physicians are known to adjust their fees downward for consumers with lower than average income when the fees are not paid by a third party. In fact, in cases of emergency, a doctor will as a rule provide medical attention with a minimum charge or no charge to a needy person. The advent of Medicaid benefits, which include physician care, did not necessarily mean more care. Instead, the physician charged fees closer to his customary level and improved his income from the same care he formerly provided at "charity" rates. Physician earnings also increased because government programs and other insurance coverage reduced the proportion of bills unpaid.

Hospital costs. Hospital daily charges rose at an average annual increase of 6.4 percent during fiscal years 1961 to 1966. In fiscal year 1967 charges rose by 16.6 percent, the rate of increase slowing only slightly during fiscal years 1968 and 1969 (15.4 percent and 14.5 percent, respectively).[51]

One study suggests that the increase in hospital costs leading to the increase in charges has not merely been the result of a rise in *prices* of inputs (wages, for example). A major portion of the increase can be accounted for by an increase in the *volume* of inputs. Hospitals have improved their facilities to meet increasing demand not only for basic services but for convenience and comfort. The rise in the prices of inputs from 1965 to 1969 was only one-third of the total rise in expenditures on hospital care. The rest of the increase was at least in part attributable to increases in volume of inputs per patient per day.[52]

It would be misleading, however, to ignore the circular nature of the rise in costs. The rise in hospital costs and medical fees up to the mid-1960s, resulting in part from the growth of third party payments under voluntary insurance, was one of the factors responsible for the institution of government insurance programs to help those who could not afford the higher costs of medical care. The counter-productive effects of these programs underline the need for careful evaluation of newly proposed programs. Extended health payments under Medicare and Medicaid were implemented at a time when the supply of facilities was inadequate to cope with the increased demand that followed upon implementation. The situation was aggravated by a time lag in building adequate facilities and training additional personnel. Moreover, as noted, the absence of advertising and other forms of rivalry such as price cutting[53] also added to the imperfections on the supply side of the market, producing monopolistic price increases.

CHAPTER III

THE NEED FOR
FEDERAL SUBSIDIES

Estimates of Medical Personnel Shortages

In 1949, the U.S. Public Health Service estimated that between 17,500 and 45,000 medical personnel were needed to bring under-served areas to an acceptable physician/population ratio. In 1953, the President's Commission on Health Needs indicated that by 1960 there would be a shortage of 59,000 physicians.[1] The Bayne-Jones Report (1958), Bayne Report (1959), and Jones Report (1960) all pointed out a shortage based on the need for maintaining the current physician/population ratio. They recommended expansion of medical school facilities and substantial federal aid both for construction and operating expenses of medical schools, and for scholarships and loans. Following these reports legislation was introduced in the 1960s to assist medical education.[2]

The figure commonly used as of 1969 for the shortage of physicians was 50,000, based on Public Health Service estimates.[3] In the hearings on the Health Professions Education Assistance Act of 1971, the method by which this was determined was given as follows: [4]

> The experience of large medical groups that provide pre-paid medical care to specified and selected populations suggests that comprehensive family health services for a population of 100,000 can be provided by 100 physicians. Application of this ratio results in a need for 12,000 physicians in the 27 States that have less than 100 physicians (private practice and full-time hospital staff, excluding psychiatrists) for every 100,000 people;
>
> 8,000 physicians to provide care in urban ghettos and other areas of special need (10 physicians for each of 800 community health centers serving 10,000 people);

15,000 psychiatrists;

10,000 physicians to fill vacancies in hospital internships and residencies; and

5,000 physicians in teaching, research, and administration, including 1,700 medical school faculty positions that are now budgeted but not filled.

This estimate appears to be relatively conservative for the following reasons:

The ratio of 100 physicians per 100,000 population is based on an effective organization of medical services for a relatively healthy section of the population.

Residents of inner cities and other low-income areas tend to be ill more often, and to have more serious illness, than more affluent populations.

No allowance is made for replacing any of the 14,500 foreign-trained physicians now serving as interns and residents in hospitals in the United States.

Requirements for additional physicians to teach students in the health related professions and occupations are growing. In recent years, faculties have been increasing, but vacancies remain high. Meanwhile, new schools of the health and allied health professions are opening, and existing schools are expanding enrollment.

Staffing requirements for public-health physicians for the administration of community health institutions, agencies, and programs are rising. Health agencies have substantial needs; and medical administrators are needed in Federal programs, hospital administration, prepayment organizations, and union health-and-welfare programs.

As long as physicians have a high degree of freedom to practice where they choose, it cannot be assumed that those added to the supply will practice in areas of greatest need.

The use of this method of estimating yields a requirement for 371,000 physicians in 1970 and 413,000 in 1980.

Other methods of estimating the shortage are quoted below from the hearings:

A second method of estimating requirements for physicians is to assume that the country as a whole should have a physician to population ratio at least equal to the highest level existing in the nine geographic divisions of the United States as defined by the Bureau of the Census. The Middle Atlantic division (consisting of New Jersey, New York, and Pennsylvania) has the highest such ratio and this results in an estimated requirement of 392,000 physicians in 1970 and 436,000 in 1980.

A third approach is to use the highest State ratio as a desirable goal. The State ratio of active physicians to population is highest in New York. There is no consensual evidence available that this State has more physicians than the numbers necessary to provide quality care to its citizens. Use of the highest State ratio produces an estimated requirement for 478,000 physicians in 1970 and 532,000 in 1980.

Other estimates of need have been developed on other bases including economic and income analyses by the Bureau of Labor Statistics, Department of Labor, that project increasing needs for physicians' services and physicians to provide them that are similar to the estimates derived from the first method of estimating outlined above.

When the supply of physicians is projected to 1980 (see Table 6) *without reference to the 1971 legislation*, the 1969 estimated shortage of 50,000 (and the 1971 shortage of 43,000) becomes a surplus of 3,000. This is with requirements defined on the basis of the Public Health Service approach (current physician/population ratio). The projected 1980 shortage is 20,000 with the requirement defined as the physician/population ratio of the highest geographic division.

Table 6

PHYSICIANS: ESTIMATED SUPPLY AND REQUIREMENTS
1970-1980

	Estimated Supply		Estimated Requirements Based On—		
Year	Pipeline	Administration proposal	1969 shortage of 50,000	Highest geographic ratio	Highest state ratio
1970	323,000	323,000	371,000	392,000	478,000
1971	332,000 a	332,000	375,000	396,000	483,000
1972	341,000	341,000	379,000	400,000	488,000
1973	350,000	350,000	383,000	404,000	493,000
1974	358,000	358,000	387,000	409,000	498,000
1975	367,000	370,000	391,000	413,000	503,000
1976	376,000	381,000	395,000	417,000	509,000
1977	386,000	394,000	399,000	422,000	514,000
1978	396,000	406,000	404,000	426,000	520,000
1979	406,000	418,000	408,000	431,000	526,000
1980	416,000	430,000	413,000	436,000	532,000

a At the end of 1971, there were 344,823 physicians on record with the American Medical Association.

Source: U.S. Congress, House of Representatives, *Health Professions Assistance Amendments of 1971, Hearings before the Subcommittee on Interstate and Foreign Commerce,* 92d Congress, 1st session, 1971, p. 943.

With the requirement defined as the ratio for the highest state, the projected shortage is 116,000.

The 1971 legislation will increase the output of physicians starting in 1975. The annual increment (net increase) in the total supply of physicians, instead of reaching 10,000 in 1980, as it would have without the 1971 legislation, will reach 12,000. This is more than twice the annual increment in physicians needed. With the effects of the 1971 legislation included, the shortage (defined by the ratio of the highest geographic division) would be eliminated by 1981; without it, the shortage by this criterion would be eliminated by the mid-1980s in any case.

If these projections are correct, the shortage of physicians is a short-run problem on the way toward solution without need for the measures adopted in 1971. The key assumption in the projections is that the annual net increase in physicians will be 9,000, rising to 10,000 in the later part of the decade. This assumes continuing inflows of foreign-trained physicians. Another assumption is the population projection, which now appears too high and which results therefore in an overestimate of physician requirements.

The projections in Table 6 are already proving too conservative. The number of physicians in 1972 was nearly 13,000 higher than projected; medical school applicants accepted for the 1972-73 freshman class were estimated at 13,500. The number of physicians, which increased by 20,000 between 1969 and 1971, will be increasing somewhat faster than projected. And projected needs for medical care must be revised downwards slightly to reflect the reduced birth rate. Thus, the 50,000 shortage could be eliminated by 1976; the shortage defined in terms of the physician/population ratio in the highest geographical region could be eliminated by 1979. Thereafter, there will be a growing surplus.

The question raised by the projections is the appropriateness of any long-term approach which permanently increases the capacity of professional schools (a capacity already more than large enough to eliminate the shortage eventually) to deal with a problem which appears on its way to disappearance. We may soon have a chronic surplus of physicians as a consequence of these federal programs and an enormous overuse of medical resources as surplus doctors try to generate a demand for their service.

There is no assured optimum physician/population ratio and no assurance that a ratio appropriate today would be appropriate ten years from now. It is unrealistic to discuss the problem solely in terms of physician/population ratios, as though other kinds of medical personnel did not count.

The second key member of the health team, the nurse, is also in short supply. The total number of registered nurses required by 1980 has been projected to be about 1 million, some 50 percent above the 660,000 employed in 1968.[5] The in-and-out movement within the profession, as a result of marriages and temporary retirement, poses an additional problem of replacement. However, a rapid increase in numbers has already substantially eliminated shortages in many areas.

The training and employment of paramedical, ancillary, or support personnel has been increased in an attempt to alleviate the shortage of doctors and nurses. The U.S. Public Health Service projects an additional need to increase these support workers by 72 percent by 1980 (1968 levels as a base) to meet the expected increase in demand for medical care. The total number required in the allied professions is said to be 250,000.[6]

Estimates of shortages of nurses and other medical personnel, based on the same approaches used for estimating shortages of physicians, rest on the assumption that the appropriate number of nurses can be determined without reference to the number of doctors, paramedics, and so on, or that the ratio of doctors to nurses implicit in whatever benchmark defines the shortage (U.S. average or ratio in state with highest ratio of physicians to population or whatever) is the proper ratio. The possibility of changing the proportions of various types of medical personnel, which would affect the estimates of shortages, will be considered in a later chapter.

Estimates of Shortages—Definitional Problems

The usual projections assume fixed ratios of medical personnel and facilities and unchanged productivity of health services. They ignore the impact of research and innovation on productivity and the possibility of substituting less expensive inputs (e.g., nurses, physician's assistants) in certain phases of the physician's activities. They also assume that prices will remain relatively unchanged; a change in the price of medical care through a restructuring of third party payments could of course alter utilization of medical care services.

The various measures of shortage used are generally based on "need" rather than on consumer demand in the economist's sense of the word. One estimate is actually a shortage from what ought to be according to the standards of the health profession. Another, deriving shortage from the standards of rich states, reflects notions of equity in the distribution of health care and services. In addition, there are conceptual definitions which lack the virtue of easy quantification. Without agreement on a definition of the proper supply, estimates of shortage are meaningless.

Definition of needs (I). One test of the adequacy of medical personnel is a technological one—a supply adequate to provide medical services to all who would benefit from them regardless of cost, regardless of how small the benefit, and regardless of the neglect of health maintenance by other means which would be caused by a diversion of resources to the provision of medical services. This may be described as the "needs" approach, and is, of course, affected by the state of the medical arts. To define a shortage on this basis, one must first define health and disease, and determine what departures from health are subject to amelioration through medical care. The need for medical care will grow as medicine widens the scope of effective treatment, even though health may improve. The medical care mix also changes: cancer and gall stones, for example, now have treatments other than surgery. Perhaps the most important issue, quite unsettled, concerns mental illness: how is it defined and diagnosed; what conditions and what individuals are treatable with any probability of measurable improvement as a result of treatment? The answers to these questions will strongly affect the order of magnitude of requirements for psychiatrists.

Definition of needs (II). Sometimes a different concept of "needs" is used in defining requirements: the supply of medical personnel which would satisfy individual demands for medical services on the assumption that services are free to the individual. This, at the limit, assumes complete insurance coverage for medical care, with initiative in the hands of the patient.

Other definitions of need. A third test is the market test—what is needed is a supply adequate to provide services demanded on a fee-for-service basis under competitive conditions. Many people needing medical care by any objective criterion would be without it under this concept. The whole thrust of legislation has therefore been away from this. The pure market test is now modified by the existence of third party payments which both increase demand and redistribute it.

A fourth test of need involves productivity of medical services. The supply should be adequate to provide all medical services for which the benefits at least equal the costs. Measuring costs is not easy, but even so it is easier than estimating the benefits from medical care.

By the criterion of consumer need or desire, regardless of price, there is a great shortage. This shortage probably cannot be eliminated. By the technological criterion of need, there is a somewhat smaller shortage. By one variety of market test, ". . . a shortage exists when the quantity of physicians' services supplied increases less rapidly than the quantity demanded at incomes received by physicians in the recent past. Under such conditions, the income of physicians relative to the income of others will tend to rise."[7] It is clear that there is a shortage and that it has worsened according to a number of measures.

First, in many areas, there are delays in getting an appointment to see a physician for anything except an emergency, delays in the doctor's waiting room even when one has an appointment, and difficulty in obtaining care at night or on weekends. Second, the incomes of physicians have risen far more rapidly than the incomes of other professionals in recent years. For the shortage (in this sense) to be eliminated, either prices would have to rise enough to eliminate delays in obtaining medical care, or supply would have to expand sufficiently to accomplish the same purpose. The first process retains restriction of supply, is made extremely unlikely by the growth of third party payments, and entails excessive earnings for physicians. The second is the only true market equilibrium, with medical care accessible to all who are willing and able to pay a price which is competitive through an unrestricted adjustment of the supply of medical services to market conditions.

By productivity criteria, there may not be a shortage, though there is maldistribution; there could even be a surplus. Whether there is a surplus, and how large, depends on valuation of benefits. That, by productivity criteria, there is no shortage is suggested by the lack of correlation between the ratio of medical personnel to population by state and indices of health and mortality. Also, apparently superior health and longevity in a number of countries with a lower ratio of medical personnel to population than the United States suggests there is no shortage here. The U.S. may already be over-doctored. This subject will be discussed in the final chapter.

Present Sources of Supply of Medical Manpower

Most of the medical manpower in the United States is provided by graduates of American and Canadian medical schools. This is not so much the case, however, of the increase in medical manpower in recent years.

The number of U.S. medical school graduates has increased by 23 percent since 1963, with 1,764 more physicians graduating in 1971 than in 1963, the year in which the Health Professions Act was enacted. Enrollments in schools of medicine and osteopathy have increased by 2,770 students, about 30 percent.[8] There are no accurate data on the number of U.S. citizens who go abroad for medical education and return to the United States to practice. It has been estimated, however, that between 500 and 600 Americans enter foreign medical schools each year. A 1969 survey showed 2,343 Americans enrolled in 16 such schools, and 162 graduated that year.[9] There is no information on the number of graduates of U.S. medical schools who emigrate, although it is believed to be insignificant.

The number of physicians known to be in active practice increased by 20 percent between 1963 and 1970.[10] In 1959, only 8.6 percent of the 241,036 physicians in the United States were graduates of foreign medical schools. By the end of 1969, 18.4 percent of the 324,942 physicians on record with the American Medical Association were graduates of foreign medical schools.[11]

Although graduates of foreign medical schools account for less than one-fifth of the total U.S. *stock* of physicians, it appears that graduates of foreign medical schools, most of whom are foreigners, accounted for about 46 percent of the *increase* in practicing physicians between 1959 and 1969. Foreigners now fill about one-third of all hospital internships and residencies. In 1951, there were just over 2,000 foreign graduates of foreign medical schools in internships and residencies, about 10 percent of the total. The number quadrupled by 1959, and the proportion rose to 23 percent. By 1969, the number rose to 14,500, and the percentage to 32.[12] A significant part of the increase in nurses and paramedical personnel in recent years has been provided by immigrants, although no specific numbers are available.

In light of the role of immigration, and of foreign medical schools as a source of supply, it is surprising that legislative attention has focused almost exclusively on the expansion of domestic capacity, though there is now some provision for assistance to Americans attending foreign medical schools. This focus is all the more surprising considering the estimates of a large current shortage, the impossibility of expanding medical school output sufficiently to eliminate the shortage quickly, and the risks inherent in rapidly increasing capacity to provide graduates who may in the long term become supernumerary. It would be possible to expand supply more quickly through utilization of capacity in foreign medical schools and through immigration, without undertaking long-term commitments. The attrition rate among immigrants would be higher than among U.S. citizens and would be more responsive to changing market conditions for doctors. This expansion route would not saddle the industry with a domestic training capacity which may prove excessive. Immigration will dwindle once the shortage is eliminated. Mothballing surplus medical schools will be more difficult.

Some consideration might be given to allowing medical services that require prolonged hospitalization or intensive care to be provided to Americans who wish them in the nations which are exporting medical personnel to the United States, or in nations such as Israel that have a surplus of doctors. In many cases, price differences are large enough to justify the transportation costs.

Maldistribution of Supply

The need to subsidize the training of professional medical manpower has been questioned. Moreover, if there is such a need, it must still be asked what phases of medical training should be subsidized. In speaking of the shortage of medical personnel, the basic emphasis is usually placed on the physician to population ratio, but this emphasis could be misleading in the aggregate. There is not so much a need to increase the ratio of physicians to population as to correct the maldistribution of physicians by specialties and geographical areas.

Maldistribution by Geographical Areas. While it may be difficult to set criteria for an efficient size of geographical area and population for delivery of health care, it is still true that there exists a maldistribution of physicians. Either in terms of "need" (as defined by social and medical criteria) or in terms of willingness to purchase more medical care at existing prices, some areas are truly underserved.

Omitting the District of Columbia, whose high physician/population ratio reflects its role as central city for a metropolitan area outside its bounds, the difference in ratio of physicians to population ranges from 238 per 100,000 in New York to 78 per 100,000 for Alaska and Mississippi—in other words by a factor of three (see Appendix Table 1). The difference in ratio of nurses to population ranged, in 1966, from 536 per 100,000 for Connecticut to 133 in Arkansas—by a factor of four (see Appendix Table 2).

Generally the wealthy states are high in both ratios, and the poorer states low in both. There are some notable exceptions. Some states, among them wealthy ones such as Alaska, with a small and dispersed population, are low in physicians and high in nurses. One might mention the Dakotas, Montana, and Wyoming in addition to Alaska. Obviously, these states substitute nurses for physicians, a point which can be proved by calculating the ratio of nurses to physicians. This is 1.9 for the nation as a whole, but 4.4 for Alaska, 3.5 for North Dakota, and 3.8 for New Hampshire. The poorer states, among them some with a fairly dispersed population, do not appear to be doing this. The ratio of nurses to physicians is below the national average for most of them, being only 1.5 for Arkansas and Tennessee and 1.6 for Texas and Oklahoma.[13]

The ratio of hospital beds to population ranges by a factor of about three. It is lowest for Alaska, with 2.1 hospital beds per thousand population, and highest for North Dakota, with 6 beds per thousand. Both of these states have unusual demographic compositions, which may help explain their extreme positions. Eliminating these outliers reduces the range to a factor of 1.9.

The tendency of physicians to concentrate in urban areas and generally in centers of knowledge and activity is natural. They stay close to centers of activity not only because of the higher income they receive there, but also because of the benefits of professional interaction and the fear of obsolescence, because of the opportunities for continuing education and growth, and the accessibility of research and modern facilities and equipment. Also, the availability of nonprofessional amenities—opportunities for recreation, education for children, cultural activities and so on—plays a role.[14]

Given the nature of physician pricing, serving in a high-income area also means higher monetary returns, although this has been modified by Medicare and Medicaid. A physician in a rural area not only serves a population with lower income, but in addition, he may face higher operating costs because of the small size of his market and difficulties in financing his investment in equipment (or even housing). He may also work longer hours to make a desirable income and to serve the needs of the community. One study suggests that physicians in rural areas work longer hours or render more service than physicians in urban areas.[15]

The average age of a physician serving in rural and isolated areas has risen from year to year. The rural physician has generally been in practice in the area for years. If he dies he frequently is not replaced. According to the Department of Agriculture, the decrease in doctors in isolated rural areas between 1950 and 1960 was six times greater than the decrease in population. The ratio of physicians to population in isolated rural areas was only one-third the national average.[16] In 1970 there were 132 counties in the nation with no doctors. Some of these counties are of course small and (in this age of improved transportation and communication) could possibly be served by a team serving several communities rather than by resident physicians and nurses.[17]

Perhaps an explanation why physicians with rural backgrounds do not return to practice in their hometowns can be gleaned from the following excerpt:

> Though there are some 43 black medical and dental students from Mississippi in various schools across the country, less than 10 percent are expected to return to the State to practice their profession. Too many of them are haunted by the memories of their family physician back home—the middle-aged, too elderly, solo practitioner who is the only black physician in a four to five county area— isolated from his colleagues and devoid of ready consultation services. They are reluctant to set up practice in an area where the mean family income among his prospective patients may run as low as $600 per year and his average working day is 16 to 18 hours long, seven days a week.[18]

It would be wrong to conclude that the overwhelming factor that keeps young doctors from returning to their hometowns is self-interest. It would be fairer to consider the practical aspect: young doctors have to repay loans incurred during their medical schooling and are saddled with these repayments while setting up practice. Later, prolonged separation may have dulled their attachment to their old hometown. New attachments may keep them in the big city.

While inaccessibility of modern facilities and opportunities for professional growth may not be the reasons for the shortage of physicians in inner cities, the quality of life there is. Moreover, until the advent of Medicaid, a practice among the low-income inner city population was also less lucrative than practice elsewhere.

Added to the socioeconomic factors that bias distribution of physicians is the impact of Flexner Report standards and quotas on the supply of Negro doctors after 1910. These standards resulted in reduction of the number of Negro medical colleges from seven in 1910 to two in 1913, aggravating the maldistribution problem.[19]

Maldistribution Among Specialties. The maldistribution of physicians among specialties aggravates the overall shortage. While general shortages exist in family or primary care medicine and some of the specialties, there is an oversupply of general surgeons.[20]

With increased demand for medical care there came a rise in the number of specialists. A former president of the American Academy of General Practice is quoted as saying that a well-trained family doctor can "comfortably and effectively care for 85 percent of the usual ordinary illnesses that beset mankind."[21] He also pointed out that only 15 percent of today's American graduates are trained to become family physicians. The trend obviously has been toward specialization. It would be helpful to know how many physicians who start out as general practitioners take further training in order to become specialists.

The ratio of general practitioners to population has been declining. In 1931, 75 percent of the physicians in the United States were general practitioners providing health care primarily outside hospitals. In 1970 only 17.6 percent of the total physician population was engaged in the practice of general medicine.[22] In 1949, the number of general practitioners per 100,000 population was 64.7; by 1967 this number had declined to 31.8. By contrast, the number of full-time specialists per 100,000 population, from 37.2 in 1949, rose to 64.7 in 1967.[23] The figures, however, are not truly comparable. The AMA included part-time specialists under the category of general practitioners before 1963. After that year, it only distinguished between specialists and general practitioners. It has not explained where those who were formerly classified as part-time specialists are now included. Also, internal medicine, although closely identified with general medicine, is treated as a specialty.[24]

In 1959, earnings of general surgeons exceeded those of general practitioners by 39.5 percent; this gap narrowed to 20.3 percent in 1970.[25] In absolute dollar amount, the gap is near $8,000 annually in both years. The gap between the earnings of internists and general practitioners widened in absolute terms (from $2,300 in 1959 to $3,850 in 1970). The highest receipts were received by specialists.

The system of closed hospital staffs tends to encourage specialization. Graduating interns know it is easier for specialists to become attached to a good hospital than for GPs.[26] The fact that specialists are favored by federal research programs also serves to entice interns away from general practice.

Among the specialties there is also maldistribution. It is generally acknowledged that while there is a shortage of radiologists and psychiatrists, there is an oversupply of surgeons. Cornell's vice president for medical affairs, Dr. Hugh Luckey, is quoted as saying that there are more neurosurgeons in New York City than in the whole of the Soviet Union, and "you have 700 times as great a chance of having your head opened up here as you would in some other countries where the quality of care is also high."[27]

A statement whose sense is repeated in different forms in different sources does not spare the profession:

> Many general surgeons are not very busy and therefore a great amount of unnecessary surgery is performed. The

situation is particularly shocking when hysterectomies are considered. We were told that many women undergo mastectomies when a less radical procedure would do. Many thyroidectomies are performed when psychotherapy would be preferred.

There is substantial overdoctoring for a host of diseases, including in particular infections of the upper respiratory tract.[28]

Not only does the overall supply of physicians influence total demand for their services, but also the distribution by specialty itself alters the structure of demand, and maldistribution by specialty tends to persist.

Are Subsidies Necessary? 1783156

The evidence is overwhelming that the $3 billion subsidy legislated in 1971 is not necessary to assure an adequate supply of medical personnel in the long run. The existing shortage is rapidly on its way to elimination without it. There is strong evidence that the subsidies legislated between 1963 and 1970 were greater than was necessary to achieve their purpose in the long run.

At no time in the last fifty years has there been a shortage of qualified applicants to medical school. No shortage is anticipated in the foreseeable future. It has been and is now possible to expand enrollment and increase the number of graduates substantially without reducing quality. Nearly all the increase in supply has taken place without the help of direct federal subsidies. Subsidies started in 1963 and could affect the supply of physicians only after a lag of several years. The present and past levels of subsidy have been in excess of the amounts needed (if any were needed) to ensure present levels of medical school graduates. A large proportion of the incremental supply—foreign-trained physicians—did not benefit from medical school subsidies. Medical school capacity and output were already being increased without the additional subsidies voted by the Congress in 1971.[29]

By a wide margin, the physician is the highest earning professional in the United States. Median earnings have increased rapidly in the last seven years. They are now in excess of $40,000. Unsubsidized loans for medical study are generally available. Nearly all entrants into medical school finish, and nearly all graduates practice medicine. There is no unemployment problem for physicians.

To summarize: (1) there is a surplus of qualified applicants to medical schools willing and able to pay the price; (2) there is an unknown number of qualified applicants willing and able to pay a

35

higher price than currently charged; (3) with high physician earnings and low attrition rates for medical students, it is feasible to finance medical education through student loans; (4) on the basis of high medical earnings, equity alone would demand that the M.D. pay the cost of his education. *It is not equitable that the highest paid profession should also have the highest training subsidy.*

The present capacity and output of medical schools will, in time, eliminate shortages by almost any definition. There is no need for further increases in the long-term capacity of medical education and output of new doctors. How quickly the shortage will be eliminated and how much surplus will develop depends on immigration policy.

CHAPTER IV

THE SCOPE FOR MORE EFFICIENT USE OF RESOURCES

The widespread concern about the inadequate supply of medical services and facilities is largely the outcome (a) of the great increase in demand for medical services resulting from the growth of third party payments; (b) of considerable misallocation of medical resources and facilities by area, by specialty, by levels of skill, and by patient; and (c) of an attitude toward the need for medical care which leads to overuse of marginal procedures.

Given all the existing barriers to the efficient use of medical resources, there is a shortage of many varieties of medical personnel and facilities. The need to increase the supply depends first on the inability or unwillingness of the medical care industry to promote efficiency and second on the criterion we use to determine an adequate supply of medical personnel and facilities.

A criterion of consumer sovereignty with third party payment would perpetuate many of the present inefficiencies and would require a large increase in supply of medical personnel. Although there are considerable differences in the ratios of doctors to population among states, there is a shortage of medical personnel even in the states with the highest ratios, according to the criterion of consumer demand. This is shown by the fact that prices tend to be higher, and physician earnings greater, in some of the states with the most doctors. The virtue of consumer sovereignty is somewhat tarnished by a system for payment of medical expenses which separates costs borne by the individual from services and benefits received by the individual. Consumer sovereignty is also questionable in an industry where the supplier—the M.D.—dominates consumer choice.

If the federal government is to continue to increase the supply of medical services by means of national subsidies, then criteria other than unqualified consumer choice should be used: criteria of national health benefits or national productivity gains. By these criteria, the case for increasing the supply of medical personnel is greatly weakened, and that for improving its allocation and productivity strengthened correspondingly. Improved allocation to underserved areas and to medical conditions whose treatment has high payoff will increase productivity. Even with a constant allocation of medical care, there are possibilities for improved productivity through greater use of paramedical personnel and reorganization of the delivery of medical care services.

Efficiency in medical care may be sought at three different levels. These are allocative efficiency, benefit-effectiveness, and cost-effectiveness.

(1) Allocative efficiency involves using available medical and health resources in those places, for those patients, in the treatment of those conditions, where medical resources are most effective. This means decreased emphasis on the old in favor of the young, on irreversible degenerative conditions in favor of acute but reversible conditions, on minor ailments which ordinarily disappear in time without medical attention in favor of those whose final outcome can be significantly influenced by treatment. This concept of efficiency runs counter to political decisions, which have stressed the needs of the old at the expense of the young, and contrary to consumer choice under third party payment systems, which allocate scarce medical resources on the basis of demand to trivial as well as to serious conditions.

(2) Benefit-effectiveness involves improving the performance of doctors and other health personnel and resources in the treatment of given conditions, primarily through better information and better diagnosis and treatment procedures. This is the principal objective of medical education and of research and development in the health field.

(3) Cost-effectiveness involves the narrowest concept of efficiency, in which for a given technology and supply of medical resources, an attempt is made to reduce the resources required to achieve a given outcome. This is particularly important in the short run, when resources are fixed and scarce. The particular resources which are scarcest, whether they be medical specialists or a particular piece of equipment or a new drug, will be used sparingly, on the basis of priorities of some kind.

Improved allocative efficiency or cost-effectiveness unequivocally reduces the shortage of medical personnel. The impact of improved benefit-effectiveness is less certain.

Problems of Productivity Measurement

To recognize the different elements that produce the final product of good health it is necessary to consider the value to the health team of other health workers, rather than focusing exclusively on the number of physicians. The shortage which legislation is supposed to remedy is actually a shortage in achievement of the desired level of health. It is identified as being the result of a shortage in the delivery of health care. If this is so, the answer may not lie in increasing doctors but in increasing the productivity of the present supply of doctors and medical facilities.

Assuming no increase in physicians, an increase in productivity would result in more services rendered per person.[1] Productivity could be improved by a better organization of the delivery of health care. As one analyst put it:

> If progress can be made in the better use and management of medical facilities, resources and personnel through functionally structured hospital services, ambulatory care, laboratory services, home care, nursing homes, public infirmaries, paramedical personnel and group practice that would increase the "productivity" of the individual physician by even 5 to 10 percent, which is conservative, the results in savings of medical manpower would offset to a considerable degree the urgent need for new medical schools.[2]

Output is difficult to measure in the health care area. There are no set relations between inputs and outputs, nor is there a satisfactory index to measure the levels of health in a given geographical area or segment of population. The problem of relating input to output is difficult not only because of the complexity of each type of care, but also because of rapid improvements in technology. Changes in medical technology have been identified as the principal cause of the decrease in the U.S. death rate from 1925 to 1960.[3]

The difficulty in measuring output and productivity makes it difficult to measure the benefits to be derived from an increase in the supply of doctors and auxiliary personnel against the cost of subsidizing this increase. Productivity in the care of a human being is an elusive concept. Results are not always directly related to the

39

quantity of inputs of knowledge and technology. There is the question of efficient manning through group practice and the efficient employment of auxiliary personnel. This efficiency can bring with it impersonality. There is no way to measure the productive effects of the closer personal relationship that exists between a solo practitioner, especially the family practitioner or internist, and his patients. Some complaints have been treated with little success because the doctor is unable to detect nonphysical factors that are hindering his success with the patient.

The higher ratio of specialists to population relative to that of general practitioners to population has other implications for the efficient use of resources. One study notes that there is substantial evidence of over-prescribing, over-hospitalizing, over-testing, and overuse of surgery.[4] After the institution of Blue Shield there were four times more tonsillectomies performed, and twice as many appendectomies, mastectomies, and hysterectomies as before. While these may have been necessary even before they were made available by insurance coverage, they also reflect the abundance of specialists available to perform them and suggest a possible misuse of resources. The study also notes that there may be more than a desirable overcapacity in the field of surgery. Whenever existing resources are underutilized and whenever there is excess capacity, productivity is lowered.

The goal should be not to increase physicians per se, but to support a policy to improve efficiency in medical care. An increase in providers of primary care (generally ambulatory or outpatient care) would improve efficiency.[5] An increase in surgeons and in other hospital-oriented specialists would only mean a continuation of the present trend of rising hospital costs and overutilization of hospital resources and specialist's care, especially since the present structure of insurance coverage by its nature encourages hospital care utilization.

Ways to Improve Productivity of the Health Care System

Allowing for difficulties in measuring qualitative effects of a change in the present system, including de-emphasizing the physician as the central figure, the following steps may be suggested as ways to increase the output of the present health care system without increasing the number of medical graduates:

(1) Redefining health service tasks so that more functions can be delegated to personnel with less training than physicians; related to this would be permitting nurses to make house calls in medically

supervised home health programs. In addition, there may be a need to review the medical degree program requirements and to develop programs for promotion from within the ranks of the medical system that involve supplementary education and training and capitalize on practical training and experience.

(2) Grouping health personnel (physicians and others) in organized settings and centralized locations so that they can share and make full use of auxiliary personnel and equipment. Related to this would be the establishment of community health centers, diagnostic clinics, and specialist group practices, as well as hospital-based group practices, regional networks, and rural health teams.

(3) Creating closer linkages between related hospitals to permit grouping of maternity, open heart surgery, and other specialized low-use services at fewer larger hospitals.

(4) Self-help units in hospitals.

(5) Automation and multiphasic screening.

(6) Intensified health education.

(7) Reducing interstate disparities in availability of medical personnel.

Redefining Health Services Tasks to Utilize Paramedical Personnel.

Although the past two decades have seen a rise in the use of auxiliary personnel in health occupations,[6] in part because of changes in medical technology and the gravitation of medical care toward institutions, the idea of a physician's assistant or nurse professional has not gained wide acceptance. At least two points need to be clarified by those who are in a position to institute changes in the system. First, are there tasks that the physician now does that do not require his highly specialized training and which others properly trained can do just as well or better with fewer years of general medical education? Second, what tasks can be undertaken by someone with less advanced general medical education under normal conditions but would require a physician's care in complex cases, and how feasible would delegating such tasks be?

The employment of additional allied health personnel to take over duties that can be delegated, if it would not have adverse impact, would leave the physician free to employ his time more efficiently. Duties that are his by their nature and not merely by rule, which could not be exercised efficiently by someone without his education and training, would be his province. Examples would be the use of midwives for normal delivery,[7] the use of nurses to administer routine patient care and to follow up on doctor care, or to take care of minor ailments.

In a study conducted in Montefiore Hospital Medical Group in New York City, whose purpose was "to explore the possibilities and evaluate the effects of introducing a public health nurse into obstetric and pediatric practice, in association with a physician, and to establish the limits of the role she might play in these professional areas," it was observed after two years that, in both phases of care, there was a saving of over 50 percent of the physician's time.[8] This was the result of substitution of visits by the public health nurse for visits by physicians. In addition, besides screening patients, the nurse discussed problems, did routine examinations, and gave guidance and advice. Contrary to commonly held fears that the public may not accept substitution of care from a paramedic for care from a doctor, the patients appeared to react favorably, and in fact, chose to give increasing responsibility to the nurse. The more challenging tasks assigned the nurse also appeared to improve nurse morale. These results could have implications for general occupational satisfaction from increased responsibilities that could affect the turnover rate in the nursing profession.

Training of new types of personnel such as physician's assistants,[9] pediatric nurse associates,[10] and the nurse professional,[11] are steps in this direction. It is recognized that reeducation of the public may be necessary in certain cases so that the patient will accept care from a non-physician with as much assurance of success as he would from a physician. This is true even considering the results of the Montefiore study, for this dealt with a limited range of medical services and a nonrepresentative group of customers. The use of nurses or physician's assistants as initial contacts and referral agents or sole dispensers of medical services also runs into legal obstacles in many states. These obstacles would have to be removed before considerable delegation by physicians or division of labor could be achieved. Among the deterrents is the physician's liability for malpractice suits for services of paramedical personnel working for him, which might affect his insurability and insurance costs. The tasks which the physician or the registered nurse may delegate may be restricted by state medical societies or by hospital practice.

The use of clinical psychologists in the treatment of mental illness is often restricted by licensing as well as by insurance coverage. Although they do not have medical school training, clinical psychologists are better trained than psychiatrists in many aspects of mental illness. Yet, many insurance policies that cover treatment of mental illness will allow payment only to psychiatrists. Many states will not allow clinical psychologists to treat the mentally ill, except under the supervision of psychiatrists, despite shortages of the latter.

Delegation of tasks from medical to paramedical personnel has three objectives: to circumvent the current shortage of medical personnel, to increase the productivity of medical care, and to reduce its cost. It involves (1) increasing the supply of existing kinds of paramedical personnel, (2) training new types of paramedical personnel who can assume responsibilities beyond those assumed by existing types, and (3) changing laws and regulations to permit the performance of duties by paramedical personnel for which they are trained, or could be trained, but which currently they are not allowed to perform. Examples are the well-baby care provided by the pediatrician and attendance at normal deliveries by the gynecologist-obstetrician. Another example may be found in the rules that prevent a nurse from diagnosing and prescribing treatment for a common cold.

One study on the possible increase in physician productivity through the use of paramedical personnel estimated that the maximum number of aides that a physician could profitably employ in private medical practice is roughly twice the present average.[12] At the suggested increased level of paramedical support the average output per physician (assuming no shortening of the workweek from its present level) was estimated to be at least 20 percent above the present level. This productivity differential is equivalent to five times the annual increase in the number of practicing physicians.

The redefining of medical tasks and fuller utilization of paramedical personnel is hampered by the prevalence of the solo practice of medicine. Restructuring the delivery of medical services toward group practice and hospital-based services may be necessary for maximum utilization of paramedical personnel.

Group Practice. The idea of increasing auxiliary personnel to increase physician productivity is usually associated with group practice. Generally the group is a formal organization of several full-time physicians, with several nurses, laboratory technicians, and a clerical staff. More efficient use of personnel through division of labor and specialization inevitably results in a saving of physician's time. It would leave the physician free to undertake the tasks for which he is uniquely qualified.

A group practice may be a multi-specialty type (e.g., the Kaiser Foundation Health Plan), a single specialty type, or general practice group. It may be a partnership, corporation, association or single owner group in which the owner employs the other physicians.[13]

Usually group practice includes expense and revenue sharing. In a prepaid group practice, also sometimes called a health maintenance organization (HMO), all-inclusive medical services are provided for a fixed payment set in advance. Physicians are paid wholly or in part on a prepaid per-capita basis—in contrast to a group where physicians are remunerated on a fee-for-service basis, in addition to sharing revenues from other services rendered in the group's facilities.[14]

One study notes that the greatest potential saving in physician's time lies in the delegation of patient care tasks but that this is not often done.[15] The amount of delegation is not related to the size of the medical firm but depends upon market demand. In fact, it is often found in small size practices where there are two or three allied workers per physician, one of whom is a registered nurse. The pressure of demand on the physician's time causes him to delegate tasks to his assistants. Moreover, patients realize the problem and accept the delegation.

There are those who argue that data show no observable economies of scale [16] in the delivery of physician services in group practice nor increases in productivity of physicians.[17] Others have argued that the system of independent solo practitioners works against efficient organization of services, economies of scale and specialization, division of labor, etc.[18] While the objective of an organization is not to keep everything and everyone busy, it would seem reasonable that solo practice would involve basic inefficiencies in idle capital equipment or even idle time for auxiliary help, unless the auxiliary help performs all tasks (from bookkeeping to taking blood samples). Productivity gains may also come from spreading the heavy cost of overhead over more patients, and from opportunities for speedier consultation and professional exchange of ideas. Economies of scale may exist particularly for specialty groups which use expensive capital equipment. For example, only 3.8 percent of psychiatrists are in group practice (this specialty requiring a minimum amount of capital equipment). On the other hand, 27.1 percent of radiologists and 18.8 percent of orthopedic surgeons engage in group practice.[19]

One study shows that there are indeed economies of scale in group practice.[20] It is, of course, possible for a group practice to grow so large that diseconomies of scale would set in because of coordination difficulties, discontinuities in adjustments, managerial inefficiency, inefficient scheduling, and so on. (Tight scheduling may mean efficient use of the physician's time, but if it means a long wait for the patient, the overall cost to society may not be as low as it